INTRODUCTION

Key ethical issues arise in association with the conduct of stem cell research by research institutions in the United States. These ethical issues, summarized in detail, receive no adequate translation into federal laws or regulations, also described in this article. U.S. Federal policy takes a passive approach to these ethical issues, translating them simply into limitations on taxpayer funding, and foregoes scientific and ethical leadership while protecting intellectual property interests through a laissez faire approach to stem cell patents and licenses. Those patents and licenses, far from being scientifically and ethically neutral in effect, virtually prohibit commercially sponsored research that could otherwise be a realistic alternative to the federal funding gap. The lack of federal funding and related data-sharing principles, combined with the effect of U.S. patent policy, the lack of key agency guidance, and the proliferation of divergent state laws arising from the lack of Federal leadership, significantly impede ethical stem cell research in the United States, without coherently supporting any consensus ethical vision. Research institutions must themselves implement steps, described in the article, to integrate addressing ethical review with the many legal compliance issues U.S. federal and state laws create.

Stem cells have a capacity for self-renewal and capability of proliferation and differentiation tovarious cell lineages. They can be classified into embryonic stem cells (ESC) and non-embryonic stem cells (non-ESC). Mesenchymal stem cells (MSC) show great promise in several animal studiesand clinical trials. ESCs have a great potential but their use is still limited due to ethical and scientific considerations. The use of amniotic fluid derived cells, umbilical cord cells, fat and skin tissues and monocytes might be an adequate "ethically pure" alternative in future. Stem cells can improve healthcare by using and augmenting the body's own regenerative potential.

Regenerative medicine aims at helping the body to form new functional tissue to replace lost or defective ones. Hopefully, this will help to provide therapeutic treatment for conditions where current therapies are inadequate. Human body has an endogenous system of regeneration through stem cells, where stem cells are found almost in every type of tissue. The idea is that restoration of function is best accomplished by these cells. Regenerative medicine comprises the use of tissue engineering and stem cell technology. This book is not meant to be exhaustive but aims to highlight present and future applications of stem cells in this exciting new discipline. We will briefly discuss tissue engineering and stem cell technology including their different sources.

BASICS

a) What is tissue engineering?

In the 1970s, Dr WT Green a paediatric orthopaedic surgeon at Boston's Children's Hospital undertook many experiments to generate new cartilage by implanting chondrocytes seeded on bone spicules in nude mice. He was unsuccessful, but his experiments were among the first attempts at what we now describe as tissue engineering. He had positively concluded that with the advent of biomaterials science it would be possible to regenerate and produce new tissues by loading viable cells onto "smart" engineered scaffolds. The term "tissue engineering" was first used in 1985, by Y.C. Fung, a pioneer of the field of biomechanics and bioengineering. Fung's concept drew on the traditional definition of "tissue" as a fundamental level of analysis of living organisms, between cells and organs. The term was coined at key workshops held at the Granlibakken Resort, Lake Tahoe, California, in February 1988 and UCLA symposium in 1992. These forums recommended that tissue engineering be designated as an emerging engineering technology. The new speciality was then famously described in an article by Langer and Vacanti in Science. They wrote: *"Tissue engineering is an interdisciplinary field that applies the principles of engineering and the life sciences toward the development of biological substitutes that restore, maintain, or improve tissue function*". Since then the novel speciality has successfully expanded and excited scientists and clinicians alike.

b) What are stem cells?

In early 1960s, Ernest A. McCulloch and James E. Till started several experiments leading to the discovery of stem cells. They injected bone marrow cells into irradiated mice, nodules developed in the spleens in proportion to the number of bone marrow cells injected. They concluded that each nodule arose from a single marrow cell. Later, they obtained evidence that these cells were capable of infinite self-renewal, a central characteristic of stem cells. Thus, stem cells have two defining properties the capacity of self-renewal giving rise to more stem cells and to differentiate into different lineages under appropriate conditions. There are two main types of stem cells, embryonic and non-embryonic. Embryonic stem cells (ESC) are pluripotent and they can differentiate into all germ layers. Non-embryonic stem cells (non-ESC) are multipotent. Their potential to differentiate into different cell types seems to be more limited. The capability for potency and the relative ease to isolate and expand these cells are invaluable properties for regenerative medicine.

c) What is the stem cell niche?

Several ideas have been put forward to explain stem cell lineage and fate determination. Current research is focused on the microenvironment or "niche" of stem cells. A niche consists of signalling molecules, inter-cellular contact, and the interaction between stem cells and their neighbouring extracellular matrix (ECM). This three-dimensional (3D) microenvironment is thought to control genes and properties that define "stemness", i.e. its self-renewal and development to committed cells. Further studies on the niche might give us a better understanding on the control of stem cell differentiation. Stem cells might be appropriately differentiated cells with the potential to display diverse cell types depending on the host niche. Furthermore, stem cells implanted into a totally different niche can potentially differentiate into cell types of the new environment. For example, human neuronal stem cells produced muscle cells when they were implanted in skeletal muscle. Bone marrow cells differentiated into neuronal cells when they were transplanted into a neural environment. These finding show possible niche influence and ASC plasticity, which is the ability to dedifferentiate into cells from other lineages. This can have clinical implications for example since both liver and pancreas develop from the same embryological line, specific growth factors and culture techniques achieved the "transdifferentiation" of liver cells to islet cells. This controversially blurs further the distinction between ESCs and ASCs.

EMBRYONIC STEM CELLS

Alexis Carrel, a Nobel laureate was an innovative surgeon whose experiments with the transplantation and the repair of body organs led to advances in the field of surgery and the art of tissue culture. On 17th January 1912 in one of his experiments he placed part of chicken's embryo heart in a fresh nutrient medium. Every 48 hours the tissue doubled in size. This continued for thirty-four years; outliving Carrel himself. Every January 17th, the doctors and nurses would celebrate with Carrel, singing "Happy Birthday" to the chicken tissue. Even though these cells were unlikely to be embryonic and possibly more related to cord-derived cells, this experiment showed the future potential of tissue culture.

Pluripotent ESCs can be derived from the inner cell mass (ICM) of a 5-6-day-old blastocyst. When a blastocyst implants the ICM eventually develops into a foetus (in two months' time). The surrounding trophoblast develops into placenta. In embryogenesis, the ICM develops into two distinct cell layers, namely the epiblast and the hypoblast. The hypoblast forms yolk sac, while the epiblast differentiates into three classical layers of the embryo; ectoderm, mesoderm and endoderm with potential of forming any tissue . ESCs were first described by Gail Martin in 1981. Thereafter, it took 17 years before the first human ESC line was established in 1998 at the University of Wisconsin-Madison. Since then, at least 225 human ESC lines have been created. An ESC line is defined by cell "immortality" in culture. An ESC line is created by culturing the ICM on feeder layers consisting of mouse embryonic fibroblasts or human feeder cells. Recent reports showed that ESCs can be grown without the use of a feeder layer, thus avoiding the exposure to viruses and exogenous proteins. Controlled differentiation into tissue committed cells is achieved by co-culture of ESCs with basic fibroblast growth factor or other cell types. Before their clinical use, ethical and scientific questions need to be resolved, e.g. the risk of teratoma formation and possible transmission of disease. Eventually, these cells might be introduced for treating diabetes. In 1869, Paul Langerhans as a medical student observed for the first-time beta islet cells as microscopic islands of a different structure in the pancreas. These complex mini-organs the pathological site of diabetes have always fascinated transplant and regenerative scientist not just for their complexity but also for their important clinical relevance. Soria et al. has been succeeded to introduce the human insulin gene into mouse ESCs to produce insulin and treat diabetic mice successfully. The history of the discovery of insulin is fascinating. The story of islet cell regeneration using ESCs is still nascent but might lead to breakthrough medical advances. Thus, the discovery of stem cells led us to predict that their use might impact health care more than the discovery of anaesthesia and antibiotics. However, their availability and derivation opened a Pandora's box of ethical dilemmas, including the moral status of the embryo, the sanctity of life and the long-standing accusation to scientists of tampering with the natural process of life.

a) Blastocyst source - therapeutic cloning

Europe's ethical and legal pluralism means that it is up to each Member State to legislate on status of the human embryo and on the use of stem cells. Thus, the legislation on ESCs is diverse in the European Union (EU). There is no legislation on embryo research in Italy, Luxemburg and Portugal. While currently, Finland, Belgium, the Netherlands, Sweden and the United Kingdom allow by law under certain conditions, the formation of ESCs lines from supernumerary embryos. Germany prohibits the latter; however, it allows by law importing of pre-formed ESC lines. Austria, Denmark, Poland, Slovakia, Lithuania, Malta, France, Ireland and Spain prohibit by law the formation and use of ESCs lines.

The contiguous point in the ethical debate on ESCs is the source of the blastocyst. These are currently derived from fertilised eggs in excess of in vitro fertilisation clinics. However, this source is limited, and another option is possible. Nuclear cloning (also known as nuclear transfer) involves the introduction of a nucleus from donor cell into an enucleated oocyte to generate an embryo with a genetic makeup 99.5% identical to that of the donor. Nuclear transfer was first reported by Briggs and King in 1952, the first vertebrate (frog) derived from nuclear transfer was reported in 1962 by Gurdon with nuclei derived from non-adult sources. The cloning of Dolly in 1997 was remarkable since she was the first mammal derived from an adult somatic cell.

Two types of nuclear cloning are described; this includes the controversial reproductive cloning where the generation of an infant with an equal genetic makeup to the donor cell is possible. Therapeutic cloning, on the other hand is used to generate early stage embryos that are explanted to produce ESC lines with an equal genetic make-up to the donor cell. Thus, this stem cell source has an unlimited capability for different immunocompatible tissue transplants.

NON-EMBRYONIC STEM CELLS

Non-ESCs are probably lower in the stem cell hierarchy. They are thought to have lost the pluripotent capability. However, throughout the organism's life, they maintain a multipotent differentiation potential. Non-ESCs can be derived from several sources including amniotic fluid, umbilical cord tissue and bone marrow.

a) Amniotic fluid derived stem cells

The ethical debate on ESCs fuelled a constant search for an adequate "ethically pure" source. Amniotic fluid contains several cell types derived from the developing foetus. These include cells with potential for differentiation. Anthony Atala's group at the Wake Forest Institute showed the ability to isolate multipotent stem cells from amniotic fluid. In addition, these undifferentiated cells express some embryonic stem cell markers. Therefore, they somehow represent an intermediate stage between the two. Amniotic fluid derived cells expand extensively without a feeder layer, doubling every 36 hours, retaining long telomeres for over 250 population doublings. These cells did not form teratomas in vivo. They showed the ability to differentiate into functional cells corresponding to each of the three embryonic germ layers (ectoderm, endoderm and mesoderm) giving rise to adipogenic, osteogenic, myogenic, endothelial, neuronal and hepatic cells. The ability to isolate genetically and phenotypically stable, pluripotent cells from such a widely and easily available source will positively have an impact on regenerative medicine.

b) Umbilical cord derived stem cells

Umbilical cord stem cells are non-ESC. However, they are closer to the embryo and they possibly retain some pluripotent characteristics. Stem cells can be harvested from cord blood and from cord lining. When transplanted, these cells show low immunogenicity and can even have localised immunosuppressive functions. These can be mediated by the release of HLA-G, IL-10 and TGF-β. This source of stem cells has the advantage of being normally discarded, with no morbidity to both mother and newborn. This leads to a limitless supply with the possibility of isolation of huge numbers of cells with no or few ethical considerations. These properties make them ideal for stem cell banking.

c) Bone-marrow derived stromal stem cells

Bone marrow derived stromal stem cells are also known as adult stem cells (BMSC). The word "stroma" is derived from Greek and the Oxford dictionary defines it as "anything spread or laid out for sitting on". The bone marrow stroma supports haemopoiesis and is made up of a network of fibroblast like cells. Among these stromal cells there is a subpopulation of multipotent cells able to generate the mesenchyme – the mass of tissue that develops mainly from the mesoderm of the embryo. This subpopulation of cell is known as mesenchymal stem cells (MSCs).

Bone marrow derived stem cells were isolated for the first time by Friedenstein and colleagues. They took bone marrow and incubated it in plastic culture dishes and after 4 hours they removed non-adherent cells. A heterogonous population of cell was retrieved with some adherent cells being spindle-shaped and forming foci of cells that then began to multiply rapidly. Thereafter, the group managed to differentiate the cells into colonies resembling deposits of bone or cartilage. Friedenstein's culture method was extensively studied finding that MSCs are capable of differentiating into several connective tissue cell types, including osteoblasts, chondrocytes, adipocytes, tenocytes and myocytes. Haematopoietic stem cells (HSCs) and MSCs are the two main types of multipotent ASCs present in the bone marrow. HSCs are committed to differentiate into blood cell lineages. These ASCs are characterised by different cell surface markers. These markers are used to select and enrich MSCs from populations of adherent bone marrow stromal cells.

Expanded MSCs also express HLA class-I but not HLA class-II antigens. However, none of these markers are specific for MSCs complicating the isolation of a pure MSC population. HSC and MSC reside in close contact in the postnatal bone marrow cavity from where they can be isolated. HSC in this cavity are functionally and structurally supported in haemopoeisis by the stroma including MSCs. Thus, this complex of heterogenous cells constitutes the "niche" of HSCs, the latter possibly also supporting MSCs, thus forming a "double niche". It is still speculative to quantify the exact numbers of stem cells since not all the cell surface markers have been identified. Risbud et al. reports that the possible bone-marrow MSCs number is between 1×10^4 and 1×10^6. Including bone marrow different tissues harbour and showed the possibility to isolate MSC. These include synovia, tendons, skeletal muscles and adipose tissue, including the fat pad of the knee joint.

The clinical application of these cells is varied. Soon these will be introduced in several fields which are currently experimental such as tendon and ligament injury. Despite improved procedures the recovery of these injuries is variable, especially in complex clinical situations. This leads to low quality tissue with a risk of rupture at the repair site or formation of fibrous adhesions. Several studies were conducted to study the possibility of cell-based regeneration. Cao et al. seeded with good results tenocytes onto polyglycolic acid scaffolds and then subcutaneously implanted into mice. These constructs were also used to regenerate flexor tendons in hens. However, tenocytes have limited donor site availability and require long in-vitro culture. Thus, a possible alternative is the use MSCs. Young et al. seeded MSCs onto rabbit 1 cm Achilles tendon defects, these showed good cross-sectional collagen fibre formation. Also, MSCs delivered onto a collagen carrier into rabbit patellar tendon defects showed marked improved stress levels. Clinical regeneration of a whole tendon/ligament construct might still have a long way to go, a more practical option is to augment and accelerate tendon healing following surgical repair. MSCs implanted within rabbit Achilles tendon repair sites were shown to contribute to early healing. MSCs can be also used clinically to augment healing at the bone-tendon interface after ACL reconstructions.

d) In vitro MSC differentiation

Human MSCs are usually isolated from the mononuclear layer of bone marrow after separation by density gradient centrifugation. These mononuclear cells are cultured in medium with 10% fetal calf serum, and the MSCs adhere to the tissue culture plastic, leaving small adherent fibroblast like cells. Thereafter, the cells divide and proliferate rapidly. As stated to some degree these cells can be induced to differentiate to any connective tissue cell type (multipotency). For example, incubating a monolayer of MSCs with asorbic acid, beta-glycerophosphate and dexamethasone for 2-3 weeks induces osteogenic differentiation. Several other methods are used to differentiate MSCs into condrocytes, adipocytes, myocytes and tenocytes in vitro.

e) Fat tissue derived stem cells

In 2002, Zuk et al. showed that human adipose "fat" tissue can be a source of multipotent stem cells. These cells can be differentiated in vitro into various cell lines including osteogenic, chondrogenic and neurogenic lineages. Myocytes and cardiomyocytes were also successfully obtained from fat tissue derived stem cells. Haematopoietic cells were derived using mouse adipose tissue derived stroma vascular fraction. These experiments showed a possible alternative source for cellular transplants and gave evidence of adipocyte cellular plasticity.

Fat tissue derived stem cells can be maintained in vitro for extended periods of time with stable population doublings and low senescence levels. Fat tissue is abundant, contains a large number of cells, and can easily be obtained with low morbidity at the harvest site. However, further work needs to be done to elucidate all the potential differences between marrow and fat derived stem cells. Still, the use of fat cells opens numerous and promising perspectives in regenerative medicine – "fat is beautiful once again".

f) Monocytes

Blood monocytes have been shown to de-differentiate under specific culture conditions, into cells which can proliferate and then differentiate into different cells including endothelial, epithelial, neuronal, liver like cells producing albumin, islet like cells producing insulin and fat cells or return back to monocytes. It might be that a "side population" of stem cells exists within a monocyte population. The ability to obtain and differentiate these pluripotent cells from autologous peripheral blood makes them valuable candidates for regenerative medicine.

g) Endothelial cells and vascularisation

Vascularisation is vital for tissue engineering. During the early stages of implantation, stem cells depend on oxygen and nutrient supply by diffusion. However, this is only effective within 100µm – 200 µm from the vascular supply. At least some progenitors in bone and marrow have a high capacity to survive in hypoxic conditions. It was shown that MSCs exhibit a remarkable tolerance to and are even stimulated by hypoxia, not unlike endothelial cells. However, cell labelling showed that a considerable loss of cells occurs within one week following implantation in porous cancellous bone matrices. Several methods are currently being studied to aid neo-vascularisation during tissue engineering. These include, adding angiogenic factors such as VEGF and FGF during implantation, co-transplanting with EC and, or modified implantation techniques. VEGF is a potent angiogenic factor and it was shown to aid vascularisation of TE constructs in several studies. Smith et al. showed that adding VEGF to cell seeded (hepatocytes) polymer scaffolds, showed improved vascularisation and significantly greater cell survival in vivo. Kaigler et al. showed that implantation of human MSCs and co-transplant of EC and MSCs on poly(lactide-co-glycolide) (PLGA) scaffold, led to significant increase of vascularisation when compared with scaffold alone. However, EC did not have a significant effect on vascularisation. These findings could be due to the release of VEGF from implanted MSCs .

CLINICAL APPLICATIONS

a) Bone

Bone defects due to congenital and acquired causes such as trauma, surgery and tumors may lead to extensive bone loss and defects which require transplantation of bone tissue or substitutes to restore structural integrity and function. Furthermore, the treatment of post-traumatic skeletal complications such as delayed unions, non-unions and malunions are challenging. The current "gold standard" is the use of autologous cancellous bone grafting. However, the supply of suitable bone is limited especially in osteoporotic, paediatric and oncological patients and its harvest results in additional morbidity to the donor site, leading to pain, haematoma, or infection. Allogenic bone has been used but this has minimal osteoinductive capacity, is possibly immunogenic, has a potential for disease transmission and is minimally replaced by new bone. Bone grafting is not effective in all cases. These patients are the ones who urgently need an improved alternative therapy. Most of the experimental and clinical evidence to date is supportive of the efficacy of MSCs in enhancing bone formation and healing of bone defects. This was proven by subcutaneous implantation in small animal models in mice and in small experimental osseous defects. Large animal models showed that the treatment of large bone defects with the application of MSCs on an osteoconductive carrier can be used successfully. Thus, experimental data in the field are strong enough to envisage translation to the clinic.

i) Bone Defects.

Clinically, Vacanti et al. reported with success tissue engineering of distal phalanx to replace this bone in a patient who suffered partial avulsion of the thumb, while Warnke et al. reconstructed the mandible of a patient after surgical removal using a titanium construct with incorporated bone morphogentic protein (BMP), bone blocks and MSCs. They "endocultivated" the whole construct in the latissimus dorsi of the patient before transfer to the defect area. Quarto et al. used a graft of hydroxyappatite and MSCs stabilized by external fixation in three patients to reconstruct 4 to 7 cm long bone defects with satisfactory incorporation and bone formation. These reports were successful since the constructs encompassed the fundamental principles of bone regeneration; osteogenesis, osteoinduction and osteoconduction along with final functional bonding between the host bone and substitute material which is called osteointegration. In future more, complex constructs should incorporate effective mechanical stimulation and better orchestration of neovascularisation.

ii) Fracture non-union

It is estimated that 10% of the fractures lead to non-union. Even though this is a well-known condition the pathogenesis is still a "mystery". A possible effective therapy is the use of MSCs to reactivate the fracture healing mechanism. Several techniques are in practice:

Un-selected un-expanded MSCs

Percutaneously injected autologous bone marrow without tissue culture has been tested in the clinical setting for the treatment of tibial non-union with mixed results . These inconclusive results are due to the low quantity. This is since most of the cells are HSCs and only one cell in 23,000 to one in 300,000 have the potential to form bone. Also, a substantial number of MSCs might be lost by apoptosis due to inadequate cellular attachment. This method might still have some benefit since growth factors and supporting "niche" cells are harvested and transferred with the bone marrow aspirate which could support the stem cells in their function

Selected expanded MSCs

Petite et al. showed in an animal model that tissue engineered bone using coral scaffold and culture expanded MSCs performed better than autologous bone marrow injection or scaffold alone. Similarly, other authors found better results following culture expansion. This is a better option since we are able to derive known selected cells and expand them to millions of cells by tissue culture from the original low number of cells. These stem cells can then be loaded on osteoconductive biodegradable matrices allowing for immediate "functional" cellular attachment. This leads to cellular mitogenesis with proliferation, differentiation, inhibition of apoptosis and ECM production in the required area. Hopefully, this reactivates the fracture healing mechanism by recruitment of the endogenous stem cells to osteoproduction and osteoinduction. The first prospective randomised controlled trial is currently underway at the Robert Jones & Agnes Hunt Orthopaedic Hospital in Oswestry to validate this treatment method in the clinical setting. A pilot study was already conducted on twelve patients with good evidence of callus formation and union.

iii) Osteogenesis imperfecta

Bone marrow derived MSCs might be effective for genetic disorders when injected systemically. This is due to the homing capability of these cells. These not only engraft to the host bone marrow but also to other multiple sites such as bone, cartilage, lung and spleen. This novel therapy can be used for osteogenesis imperfecta (OI), currently an untreatable genetic disorder caused by defects in the major bone extracellular matrix structural protein, type I collagen. There are six types of OI, though the symptoms range from person to person. Type I is the most common and mildest form, followed by Type II, Type III and Type IV. Types V and VI have been more recently classified, and they share the same clinical features of IV, but each have unique histological findings. Horwitz et al. used allogenic bone marrow transplantation in three children suffering from the disorder. After three months the total bone mineral content increased, fracture rate decreased, and trabecular bone showed new dense bone formation. The authors concluded that this improvement is possibly due to engraftment of transplant bone marrow derived MSCs, which generate osteoblast capable of secreting normal extracellular proteins. This study showed encouraging results, however it remains to be determined to what extent the cells contribute to the overall results.

b) Cartilage

Articular cartilage is vulnerable to injury with a poor potential for regeneration leading to early degeneration and later arthritic changes. Even though joint arthroplasties have improved considerably over the last decade, cell-based therapy to repair cartilage defects at an earlier stage is needed.

Procedures using stem cells are available; 'Microfracture' introduced by Steadman et al. leads to penetration of subchondral bone. When the tourniquet is released, possible recruitment of stem cells from the underlying bone marrow leads to the formation of a "super clot". A report shows 11% of biopsies being predominantly hyaline cartilage and 17% a mixture of fibrocartilage and hyaline. However, this technique is not adequate for large lesions and results are not always consistent. Another available therapy is autologous chondrocyte implantation (ACI) was first performed in 1987 by Peterson in Gothenburg. This leads to an alternative cell-based therapy for the treatment of chondral and osteochondral defects. In this technique differentiated chondrocytes are isolated from autologous non-weight bearing cartilage and expanded to millions of cells by tissue culture. The cells are then re-implanted into the defect under a periosteal (109) or more recently under a biodegradable membrane. Even though, chondrocytes in two-dimensional cell cultures are known to alter their phenotype and dedifferentiate to fibroblast cells losing the ability for collagen II and proteoglycan formation clinical results at 11 years follow-up are rated as good or excellent in 84% of patients. Autologous matrix induced chondrogenesis (AMIC) is a novel therapy which uses a porcine collagen I/III matrix patch over a defect which has been microfractured. This patch is supposed to keep the "super clot" contents i.e. stem cells, protected in the early post-operative stage and thus accommodate chondrogenic differentiation. When compared to ACI, AMIC avoids the need for time consuming and costly tissue culture while exploiting the stem cell potential from the subchondral bone.

The main criticism for ACI is that it requires an invasive procedure to harvest chondrocytes from adjacent intact areas. MSCs are an alternative source of cells. These can be derived from several sources such as the bone marrow and fat. Utilising MSCs and directing them into chondrogenic differentiation might lead to the formation of higher quality cartilage, that is a larger composition of hyaline, adequate structural reorganization and thus better biomechanical properties. Wakitani et al. used successfully MSCs in a type I collagen gel to repair carpine chondral defects. This was translated successfully to clinical practice. Autologous bone marrow derived MSCs transplantation was used for the repair of full-thickness articular cartilage defects in the patellae of two patients. Wakitani et al. also reported on twelve patients suffering from knee osteoarthritis (OA) who received MSCs injected into cartilage defects of the medial femoral condyle at the time of high tibial osteotomy. These were then covered by periosteum. The control group underwent the same procedure but received no cells. Although the clinical improvement was not significantly different, MSCs treated patients had better arthroscopic and histological grading scores.

Soon a novel approach for OA could be the use of MSCs to inhibit progression of the disease. In OA, it was found that stem cells are depleted and have reduced proliferation and differentiation capabilities. Thus, the systemic or local delivery of stem cells, thus, might augment the regenerative cell population and possibly induce repair or inhibit progression of the condition. Murphy et al. percutaneously injected MSCs suspended in sodium hyaluronan into a carpine OA model. It was shown that the MSCs stimulated regeneration of meniscal tissue with implanted MSCs detected in the regenerate. Degenerated cartilage, osteophytic remodelling, and subchondral sclerosis were reduced in the cell treated joints compared with the control. These experiments implicate that MSCs hold exciting promise for regenerating meniscus and preventing OA. There is a group in Singapore that uses this procedure clinically with success.

c) Cardiac Muscle

The discovery of an endogenous repair system questions the old paradigm that describes the heart as a post-mitotic organ and introduces the notion that cardiac regeneration can be regulated by stem cells. In fact, dividing cells with large mitotic figures were found in cardiac muscle. However, their proportion is very low (0.015-0.08%). The origin of these cells is uncertain. They can be endogenous, derived from the epicardium or even be extracardiac. The latter is suggested by investigations in sex-matched heart transplant patients were male patients who received female hearts showed cardiomyocyte biopsies carrying the Y chromosome. This leads us to hypothesise that circulating stem cells are homing for regeneration.

Regenerating ischaemic heart disease can be achieved by delivering culture expanded MSCs into the coronary arteries or directly into the myocardium to expand the endogenous regenerative pool.

Janssens et al. reported the first randomised controlled trial of autologous bone marrow MSCs implantation for patients with ST-elevation myocardial infarction. Stem cell therapy provided significant reductions in myocardial infarct size and better recovery rates of regional systolic function after four months follow up. However, there was no significant benefit in terms of left ventricular ejection fraction, myocardial perfusion and cardiac metabolism. In addition, there is no evidence to date that MSCs produce contractile structures in the cardiac muscle following implantation. Despite these mixed results the use of stem cells is a promising option for treating patients with acute myocardial infarction.

d) Urinary Tissues - Bladder

Urologists have always been faced with the problem of bladder replacement. Traditionally, this has been undertaken with intestinal segments. However, this involves complicated bowel resection and possible complications such as adhesions, mucus secretion, metabolic derangements and malignant transformation. Thus, an adequate alternative is needed. Cell based regeneration of bioengineered bladder has been reported in several animal models. Atala et al. reported the first clinical trial of engineered bladders in seven patients with myelomeningocele suffering from high-pressure or poorly compliant bladders.

Autologous urothelial and smooth muscle cells were cultured for six weeks, and then seeded on biodegradable 3D matrices made of collagen or a composite of collagen and polyglycolic acid (PGA). Thereafter, augmentation cystoplasty utilising the engineered construct was undertaken. Over a mean follow-up of almost four years all patients showed improved overall bladder function with no complications. The patients who had an omentum wrapped around the construct showed the best results. Most probably, the omentum was a source of neovascularisation; a vital element in regenerative medicine.

Bladder tissue engineering using MSCs might show better results than differentiate cells. MSCs were shown to migrate to the bladder grafts and differentiate into smooth muscle. These achieved fast repopulation of the grafts, exhibited appropriate neural function and showed less fibrosis. Utilising autologous bladder cells might be inadequate if bladder cancer is present. Clinical application of bladder tissue engineering made important steps. However, more needs to be done for achieving the target of whole organ regeneration and transplantation in urology.

e) Spinal Cord

Pluripotent cells can differentiate into neural tissue including neurons, astrocytes and oligodendrocytes. The presence of endogenous stem cells in the mammalian spinal cord, suggest an inherent capacity for regeneration. Animal models showed axonal regeneration and functional recovery after spinal cord injury. Akiyama et al. found that MSCs can remyelinate spinal cord axons after direct injection into the lesion. Traumatic spinal cord injury (SCI) can lead to severe neurological damage. Even though endogenous stem cells are present, recovery from this injury is difficult. A strategy to increase axonal regeneration could involve transplantation of stem cells into the injured spinal cord. Park et al. conducted a clinical study on five patients with acute SCI, these were treated by bone marrow derived cells and granulocyte-macrophage colony stimulating factor (GM-CSF). GM-CSF is a signalling molecule that induces proliferation and differentiation of bone marrow cells. Also, it possibly leads to proliferation of endogenous neural stem cells, inhibits apoptosis and activates macrophages which remove the myelin debris inhibiting regeneration. The patients showed sensory and motor function improvements with no complications. These are encouraging results. However, the extent of regeneration and to what level are the stem cell contribution is unknown. The translation of animal models to human trials is difficult and the repair of the spinal cord still very complex. Randomised controlled clinical trials are needed to understand the full picture of stem cell therapy in spinal cord injuries.

CONCLUSIONS

At present more, trials are needed to determine the exact role of stem cells in regenerative medicine. MSCs showed great promise in several animal studies and clinical trials. ESCs have a great potential due to their characteristics but their use is limited by ethical considerations. The use of amniotic fluid cells, umbilical cord cells, fat and skin tissue and monocytes might be an adequate alternative. Current laboratory and animal trials are studying the possibility of introducing stem cell therapy to clinical practice for regeneration in muscular dystrophy, intervertebral disc degeneration, cerebral infarcts and transplantation medicine. These studies show encouraging results to enable us to harness and augment under controlled conditions, the body's own regenerative potential.

References

1. Green WT Jr. Articular cartilage repair. Behavior of rabbit chondrocytes during tissue culture and subsequent allografting. Clin Orthop Relat Res. 1977 May;(124):237-50

2. "Tissue Engineering. Selected Papers from the UCLA Symposium of Tissue Engineering. Keystone, Colorado, April 6-12, 1990", J Biomech Eng 1991 May;113(2):111-207.

3. Langer R, Vacanti JP. Tissue engineering. Science 1993; 260:920.

4. Becker AJ, McCulloch EA, Till JE. Cytological demonstration of the clonal nature of spleen colonies derived from transplanted mouse marrow cells. Nature. 1963 Feb 2; 197:452-4.

5. Lee EH, Hui JHP. The potential of stem cells in orthopaedic surgery. J Bone Joint Surg 2006 July;88(7):841-853.

6. Watt FM, Hogan BL. Out of Eden: stem cells and their niches. Science 2000; 287:1427-30.

7. Wu P, Tarasenko YI, Gu Y et al. Region specific generation of cholinergic neurons from fetal human neural stem cells grafted in adult rat. Nat Neurosci 2002; 5:1271-8.

8. Galli R, Borello U, Gritti A et al. Skeletal myogenic potential of human and mouse neural stem cells. Nat Neurol 2000; 3:986-91.

9. Zhao LR, Duran WM, Reyes M et al. Human bone marrow stem cells exhibit neural phenotypes and ameliorate neurological deficits after grafting into the ischemic brain of rats. Exp Neurol 2002; 174:11-20.

10. Mezek E, Key S, Vogelsang G et al. Transplanted bone marrow generates new neurons in human brains. Proc Natl Acad Sci USA 2003; 100:1364-9.

11. Alam T, Sollinger HW. Glucose-regulated insulin production in hepatocytes. Transplantation 2002 vol.74 no.12. pp 1781-1787.

12. Witkowski JA. Dr. Carrel's immortal cells. Med Hist. 1980 Apr;24(2):129-42.

13. Martin, G.R. Isolation of a pluripotent cell line from early mouse embryos cultured in medium conditioned by teratocarcinoma stem cells. Proc. at. Acad. Sci. USA. 1981;78: 7634-7638.

14. Thompson JA, Itskovitz-Eldor J, Shapiro SS, et al. Embryonic stem cell lines derived from human blastocysts. Science 1998; 282:1145-7.

15. Richards M, Fong C-Y, Chan W-K et al. Human feeders support prolonged undifferentiated growth of human inner cell masses and embryonic stem cells. Nat Biotechnol 2002;20:933– 936.

16. Sakula A. Paul Langerhans (1847-1888): a centenary tribute. J R Soc Med. 1988 Jul;81(7):414-5.

17. Calne R. The challenges of cell-transplantation and genetic engineering for the treatment of diabetes and haemophilia. In: Ashammakhi N, Reis RL, Chelliellini E, Eds. Topics in Tissue Engineering, Vol 3. E-book http:// www.oulu.fi/spareparts/ebook_topics_in_t_e_vol3/

18. Soria B, Roche E, Berna G, Leon-Quinto T, Reig JA, Martin E. Insulin-secreting cell derived from embryonic stem cells normalize glycemia in streptozotocin-induced diabetic mice. Diabetes 2000;49(2):157-62.

19. http://ec.europa.eu/research/press/2003/pdf/sec2003-441report_en.pdf. Last Accessed on: 2/2/2007

20. Briggs R, King TJ. Transplantation of living nuclei from blastula cells into enucleated frogs' eggs. Proc Natl Acad Sci USA 1952; 38:455-463.

21. Gurdon JB. Adult frogs derived from the nuclei of single somatic cells. Dev Biol 1962; 4:256-273.

22. Campbell KH, McWhir J, Ritchie WA, Wilmut I. Sheep cloned by nuclear transfer from a cultured cell line. Nature 1996; 380:64-66

23. Priest RE, Marimuthu KM, Priest JH. Origin of cells in human amniotic fluid cultures: ultrastructural features. Lab. Invest. 1978; 39:39,106-109.

24. De Coppi P, Bartsch G, Sidddiqui MM, Xu T, Santor CC, Mostoslavsky G, Serre AG et al. Isolation of amniotic stem cell lines with potential for therapy. Nat. Biotechnology. 2007;25(1):100-106.

25. Houlihan JM, Biro PA, Harper HM, Jenkinson HJ, Holmes CH. The human amnion is a site of MHC class Ib expression: evidence for the expression of HLA-E and HLA-G. J Immunol. 1995 Jun 1;154(11):5665-74.

26. Taylor A, Verhagen J, Blaser K, Akdis M, Akdis CA. Mechanisms of immune suppression by interleukin-10 and transforming growth factor beta: the role of T regulatory cells. Immunology 2006 Apr;117(4):433-42.

27. The new shorter oxford dictionary on historical principles. Ed. Brown L. 1993; 2:3101, Calaredon press. Oxford.

28. Caplan AI. Mesenchymal stem cells. J Orthop Res. 1991 Sep;9(5):641-50.

29. Caplan AI. The mesengenic process. Clin Plast Surg. 1994 Jul;21(3):429-35.

30. Friedenstein, A. J., Petrakova, K. V., Kurolesova, A. I., & Frolova, G. P. Heterotopic of bone marrow.Analysis of precursor cells for osteogenic and hematopoietic tissues. Transplantation, 1968:6; 230-247.

31. Friedenstein, A. J., Chailakhyan, R. K., Latsinik, N. V., Panasyuk, A. F., & Keiliss-Borok, I. V. (1974). Stromal cells responsible for transferring the microenvironment of the hemopoietic tissues. Cloning in vitro and retransplantation in vivo. Transplantation, 1974:17;331-340.

32. Friedenstein, A. J. Precursor cells of mechanocytes. Int Rev Cytol, 1976:47;327-359.

33. Friedenstein, A. J., Gorskaja, J. F., & Kulagina, N. N. (1976). Fibroblast precursors in normal and irradiated mouse hematopoietic organs. Exp Hematol, 1976:4;267-274.

34. Friedenstein, A. J., Chailakhyan, R. K., & Gerasimov, U. V. Bone marrow osteogenic stem cells: in vitro cultivation and transplantation in diffusion chambers. Cell Tissue Kinet., 1987:20;263-2.

35. Friedenstein AJ, Piatetzky-Shapiro II, Petrakova KV. Osteogenesis in transplants of bone marrow cells. J Embryol Exp Morphol 1966; 16:381-390.

36. Caplan AI. Mesenchymal Stem Cells. J Orthop Res 1991; 9:641-650.

37. Dexter TM, Allen TD, Lajtha LG. Conditions controlling the proliferation of haemopoietic stem cells in vitro. J Cell Physiol 1977; 91:335-344.

38. Tavassoli M, Friedenstein A. Haemopoietic stromal environment. Am J Hematol 1983; 15:195-203.

39. Risbud MV, Sittinger M. Tissue engineering: advances in in vitro cartilage generation. Trends Biotechnol 2002;20(8):351-6.

40. De Bari C, Dell'Accio F, Vandenabeele F et al. Skeletal muscle repair by adult human mesenchymal stem cells from synovial membrane. J Cell Biol. 2003 Mar 17;160(6):909-18.

41. Salingcarnboriboon R, Yoshitake H, Tsuji K et al. Establishment of tendon-derived cell lines exhibiting pluripotent mesenchymal stem cell-like property. Exp Cell Res. 2003 Jul 15;287(2):289-300.

42. Bosch P, Musgrave DS, Lee JY et al. Osteoprogenitor cells within skeletal muscle. J Orthop Res. 2000 Nov;18(6):933-44.

43. Draggo JL, Samimi B, Zhu M et al. Tissue-engineered cartilage and bone using stem cells fromhuman infrapatellar fat pads. J Bone Joint Surg [Br]. 2003 Jul;85(5):740-7.

44. Cao Y, Vacanti JP, Ma X, Paige KT, Upton J, Chowanski Z, Schloo B, Langer R, Vacanti CA. Generation of neo-tendon using synthetic polymers seeded with tenocytes. Transplant Proc. 1994 Dec;26(6):3390-2.

45. Cao Y, Liu Y, Liu W, Shan Q, Buonocore SD, Cui L. Bridging tendon defects using autologous tenocyte engineered tendon in a hen model. Plast Reconstr Surg. 2002 Oct;110(5):1280-9.

46. Young RG, Butler DL, Weber W et al. Use of mesenchymal stem cells in a collagen matrix for Achilles tendon repair. J Orthop Res 1998; 16:406-13.

47. Awad Ha, Boivin GP, Dressler MR, et al. Repair of patellar tendon injuries using a cellcollagen composite. J Orthop Res 2003; 21:420-31.

48. Chong AK, Ang AD, Goh JC, Hui JH, Lim AY, Lee EH, Lim BH. Bone marrow-derived mesenchymal stem cells influence early tendon-healing in a rabbit achilles tendon model. J Bone Joint Surg Am. 2007 Jan;89(1):74-81.

49. Lim JK, Hui J, Li L, Thambyah A, Goh J, Lee EH. Enhancement of tendon graft osteointegration using mesenchymal stem cells in a rabbit model of anterior cruciate ligament reconstruction. Arthroscopy. 2004 Nov;20(9):899-910.

50. Colter DC, Class R, DiGirolamo CM, Prockop DJ. Rapid expansion of recycling stem cells in cultures of plastic-adherent cells from human bone marrow. Proc atl Acad Sci U S A. 2000;28;97(7):3213-8.

51. Zuk, P. A., M. Zhu, P. Ashjian, D. A. De Ugarte, J. I. Huang, H. Mizuno, Z. C. Alfonso, J. K. Fraser, P. Benhaim, M. H. Hedrick. Human adipose tissue is a source of multipotent stem cells. Mol Biol Cell 2002;13(12): 4279-95.

52. Halvorsen, Y. D., D. Franklin, A. L. Bond, D. C. Hitt, C. Auchter, A. L. Boskey, E. P. Paschalis, W. O. Wilkison, J. M. Gimble. Extracellular matrix mineralization and osteoblast gene expression by human adipose tissue-derived stromal cells. Tissue Eng 2001;7(6): 729- 41.

53. Huang, J. I., P. A. Zuk, N. F. Jones, M. Zhu, H. P. Lorenz, M. H. Hedrick, P. Benhaim. Chondrogenic potential of multipotential cells from human adipose tissue. Plast Reconstr Surg 2004;13(2): 585-94.

54. Erickson GR, Gimble JM, Franklin DM, Rice HE, Awad H, Guilak F. Chondrogenic potential of adipose tissue-derived stromal cells in vitro and in vivo. Biochem. Biophys. Res. Commun. 2002; 290:763

55. Zuk PA, Zhu M, Mizuno H, Huang J, Futrell JW, Katz AJ, Benhaim P, Lorenz HP, Hendrick MH. Multilineage cells from human adipose tissue: Implications for cell-based therapies. Tissue Eng. 2001; 7:211.

56. Safford, K. M., K. C. Hicok, S. D. Safford, Y. D. Halvorsen, W. O. Wilkison, J. M. Gimble, H. E. Rice. Neurogenic differentiation of murine and human adipose-derived stromal cells. Biochem Biophys Res Commun 2002;294(2): 371-9.

57. Ashjian, P. H., A. S. Elbarbary, B. Edmonds, D. DeUgarte, M. Zhu, P. A. Zuk, H. P. Lorenz, P. Benhaim, M. H. Hedrick. In vitro differentiation of human processed lipoaspirate cells into early neural progenitors. Plast Reconstr Surg 2003;111(6): 1922-31.

58. Mizuno, H., P. A. Zuk, M. Zhu, H. P. Lorenz, P. Benhaim, M. H. Hedrick. Myogenic differentiation by human processed lipoaspirate cells. Plast Reconstr Surg 2002;109(1): 199-209

59. Rangappa, S., C. Fen, E. H. Lee, A. Bongso, E. K. Sim. Transformation of adult mesenchymal stem cells isolated from the fatty tissue into cardiomyocytes. Ann Thorac Surg 2003;75(3): 775-9.

60. Cousin, B., Andre M, Arnaud E, Penicaud L, Casteilla L. Reconstitution of lethally irradiated mice by cells isolated from adipose tissue. Biochem Biophys Res Commun 2003;301(4): 1016-22.

61. Charriere, G., B. Cousin, E. Arnaud, M. Andre, F. Bacou, L. Penicaud, L. Casteilla. Preadipocyte conversion to macrophage. Evidence of plasticity. J Biol Chem 2003;278(11): 9850-5.

62. Zhao Y, Glesne D, Huberman E. A human peripheral blood monocyte-derived subset acts as pluripotent stem cells. PAS 2003;100(5):2426-31.

63. Ruhnke M, Ungefroren H, Nussler A. Differentiation of in vitro modified human peripheral blood monocytes into hepatocyte-like and pancreatic islet-like cells. Gastroenterology 2005;128(7):1774-86.

64. Kneser U, Schaefer DJ, Polykandriotis E, Horch RE. Tissue engineering of bone: the reconstructive surgeon's point of view. J Cell Mol Med. 2006 Jan-Mar;10(1):7-19.

65. Logeart-Avramoglou D, Anagnostou F, Bizios R, Petite H. Engineering bone: challenges and obstacles. J Cell Mol Med. 2005 Jan-Mar;9(1):72-84.

66. Lennon DP, Edmison JM, Caplan AI. Cultivation of rat marrow-derived mesenchymal stem cells in reduced oxygen tension: effects on in vitro and in vivo osteochondrogenesis. J Cell Physiol. 2001 Jun;187(3):345-55.

67. Ivanovic Z, Bartolozzi B, Bernabei PA, Cipolleschi MG, Rovida E, Milenkovic P, Praloran V, Dello Sbarba P. Incubation of murine bone marrow cells in hypoxia ensures the maintenance of marrow-repopulating ability together with the expansion of committed progenitors. Br J Haematol. 2000 Feb;108(2):424-9.

68. Nomi M, Atala A, Coppi PD, Soker S. Principals of neovascularization for tissue engineering. Mol Aspects Med. 2002 Dec;23(6):463-83.

69. Yancopoulos GD, Davis S, Gale NW, Rudge JS, Wiegand SJ, Holash J. Vascular-specific growth factors and blood vessel formation. Nature. 2000 Sep 14;407(6801):242-8.

70. Elcin YM, Dixit V, Gitnick G. Extensive in vivo angiogenesis following controlled release of human vascular endothelial cell growth factor: implications for tissue engineering and wound healing. Artif Organs. 2001 Jul;25(7):558-65.

71. Martin GR. Isolation of a pluripotent cell line from early mouse embryos cultured in medium conditioned by teratocarcinoma stem cells. Proc Natl Acad Sci U S A. 1981 Dec;78(12):7634-8.

72. Smith MK, Peters MC, Richardson TP, Garbern JC, Mooney DJ. Locally enhanced angiogenesis promotes transplanted cell survival. Tissue Eng. 2004 Jan-Feb;10(1-2):63-71.

73. Kaigler D, Krebsbach PH, Wang Z, West ER, Horger K, Mooney DJ. Transplanted endothelial cells enhance orthotopic bone regeneration. J Dent Res. 2006 Jul;85(7):633-7.

74. Kaigler D, Krebsbach PH, Polverini PJ, Mooney DJ. Role of vascular endothelial growth factor in bone marrow stromal cell modulation of endothelial cells. Tissue Eng. 2003 Feb;9(1):95-103.

75. Al-Khaldi A, Eliopoulos N, Martineau D, Lejeune L, Lachapelle K, Galipeau J. Postnatal bone marrow stromal cells elicit a potent VEGF-dependent neoangiogenic response in vivo. Gene Ther. 2003 Apr;10(8):621-9.

76. Meister K, Segal D, Whitelaw GP. The role of bone grafting in the treatment of delayed unions and nonunions of the tibia. Orthop Rev 1990; 19:2600-71.

77. Enneking WF, Campanacci DA. Retrieved human allografts: a clinicopathological study. J Bone Joint Surg Am. 2001 Jul;83-A (7):971-86.

78. Goshima J, Goldberg VM, Caplan AI. The osteogenic potential of culture-expanded rat marrow mesenchymal cells assayed in vivo in calcium phosphate ceramic blocks. Clin Orthop 1991; 262:298-311.

79. Krebsbach Ph, Kuznetsov SA, Satomura K et al. Bone formation in vivo: comparison of osteogenesis by transplanted mouse and human marrow stromal fibroblasts. Transplantation 1997; 63:1059-1069.

80. Krebsbach PH, Mnakani MH, Satomura K et al. Repair of craniotomy defects using bone marrow stromal cells. Transplantation 1998; 66:1272-1278.

81. Ohgushi H, Goldberg VM, Caplan AI. Repair of bone defects with marrow cells and porous ceramic. Experiments in rats. Acta Orthop Scand 1989; 60:334-339.

82. Kadiyala S, Young RG, Thiede MA et al. Culture expanded canine mesenchymal stem cells possess osteochondrogenic potential in vivo and in vitro. Cell Transplant 1997; 6:125-134.

83. Bruder SP, Kraus KH, Goldberg VM, Kadiyala S. The effect of implants loaded with autologous mesenchymal stem cells on the healing of canine segmental bone defects. J Bone Joint Surg [Am], 1998, 80:7 (985-996).

84. Kon E, Muraglia A, Corsi A et al. Autologous bone marrow stromal cells loaded onto porous hydroxyapatite ceramic accelerate bone repair in critical-size defects of sheep long bones. J Biomed Mater Res 2000; 49:328-337.

85. Petite H, Viateau V, Bensaid W, Meunier A et al. Tissue-engineered bone regeneration. ature Biotechnology 2000; 18:959-963.

86. Den Boer FC, Wippermann BW, Blockhuis TJ, Patka P, Bakker FC, Haarman HJThM. Healing of segmental bone defects with granular porous hydroxyapatite augmented with recombinant human osteogenic protein-1 or autologous bone marrow. J Orthop Res, 2003, 21:3 (521-528).

87. Vacanti CA, Bonassir LJ, Vacanti MP, Schufflebarger J. Replacement of an avulsed phalanx with tissue-engineered bone. Engl J Med. 2001;344,20:1511-1514.

88. Warnke PH, Springer IN, Wiltfang J, Acil Y et al. Growth and transplantation of a custom vascularised bone graft in a man. Lancet 2004 Aug 28-Sep3;364(9436):766-70.

89. Quarto R, Mastrogiacomo M, Cancedda R et al. Repair of large bone defects with the use of autologous bone marrow stromal cells. Engl J Med 2001;344:385–386.

90. Einhorn TA. Enhancement of fracture-healing. J Bone Joint surg [Am] 1005;77-A:940-56.

91. Hernigou P, Poignard A, Manicom O. The use of percutaneous autologous bone marrow transplantation in non-union and concentration of progenitor cells. J Bone Joint Surg [Br] 2005;87-B:896-902.

92. Healey JH, Zimmerman PA, McDonnell JM, Lane JM. Percutaneous bone marrow grafting of delayed union and nonunion in cancer patients. Clin Orthop. 1990 Jul (256): 280-5.

93. Hernigou P, Poignard A, Manicom O. The use of percutaneous autologous bone marrow transplantation in non-union and concentration of progenitor cells. J Bone Joint Surg [Br] 2005;87-B:896-902.

94. Goel A, Sangwan SS, Siwach RC, Ali AM. Percutaneous bone marrow grafting for the treatment of tibial non-union. Injury. 2005 Jan;36(1):203-6.

95. Bensaid W, Oudina K, Viateau V, Potier E, Bousson V, Blanchat C, Sedel L, Guillemin G, Petite H. De novo reconstruction of functional bone by tissue engineering in the metatarsal sheep model. Tissue Eng. 2005 May-Jun;11(5-6):814-24.

96. Mankani MH, Kuznetsov SA, Shannon B, Nalla RK, Ritchie RO, Qin Y, Robey PG. Canine cranial reconstruction using autologous bone marrow stromal cells. Am J Pathol. 2006 Feb;168(2):542-50.

97. Kruyt MC, Dhert WJ, Oner FC, van Blitterswijk CA, Verbout AJ, de Bruijn JD. Analysis of ectopic and orthotopic bone formation in cell-based tissue-engineered constructs in goats. Biomaterials. 2007 Apr;28(10):1798-805.

98. Bacakova L, Filova E, Rypacek F, Svorcik V, Stary V. Cell adhesion on artificial materials for tissue engineering. Physiol Res. 2004;53 Suppl 1: S35-45.

99. Bajada S, Harrison P, Ashton BA, Cassar-Pullicino V, Ashammakhi N, Richardson JB. Successful healing of Refractory Tibial Non-union by combined Calcium Sulphate and Stromal Cell Implantation. First Report. J Bone Joint Surg [Br] 2007 Oct;89(10),1382-6.

100. Pereira RF, Halford KW, O'Hara MD et al. Cultured adherent cells from marrow can serve as long-lasting precursor cells for bone, cartilage, and lung in irradiated mice. Proc Natl Acad Sci USA 1995;92:4857-4861.

101. Goan SR, Junghahn I, Wissler M et al. Donor stromal cells from human blood engraft in NOD/SCID mice. Blood 2000; 96:3871-3978.

102. Devine SM, Bartholomew AM, Mahmud N et al. Mesenchymal stem cells are capable of homing to the bone marrow of non-human primates following systemic infusion. Exp Hematol 2001; 29:244-255.

103. Horwitz EM, Prockop DJ, Fitzpatrick LA et al. Transplantability and therapeutic effects of bone marrow-derived mesenchymal cells in children with osteogenesis imperfecta. Nat Med 1999; 5:309-313.

104. Horwitz EM, Prockop DJ, Gordon PL et al. Clinical responses to bone marrow transplantation in children with severe osteogenesis imperfecta. Blood 2001; 97:1227-1231.

105. Steadman JR, Rodkey WG, Singleton SB, Briggs KK. Microfracture technique for fullthickness chondral defects: technique and clinical results. Operative Tech in Orthop 1997; 7:300-4.

106. Steadman JR, Rodkey WG, Rodrigo JJ. Microfracture: surgical technique and rehabilitation to treat chondral defects. Clin.Orthop.2001;391(Suppl): S362-9.

107. Knutsen G, Engebretsen L, Ludvigsen TC, Drogset JO, Grontvedt T, Solheim E et al. Autologous condrocyte implantation compared with microfracture in the knee. A randomized trial. J Bone Joint Surg [Am] 2004;86A:455-64.

108. Kreuz PC, Steinwachs MR, Erggelet C et al. Results after microfracture of full-thickness chondral defects in different compartments in the knee. Osteoarthrits and Cartilage 2006;14(11):1119-25.

109. Richardson JB, Caterson B, Evans EH et al. Repair of human articular cartilage after implantation of autologous chondrocytes. J Bone Joint Surg [Br] 1999; 81:1064-1068.

110. Song Y, Ma H, Cai Z. [A study on guided tissue regeneration and tissue engineeringtransplantation of collagen membrane seeded with cultured hyaline chondrocytes] Zhonghua Zheng Xing Shao Shang Wai Ke Za Zhi. 1999 May;15(3):175-7.

111. von der Mark K, Gauss V, von der Mark H, Muller P. Relationship between cell shape and type of collagen synthesized as chondrocytes lose their cartilage phenotype in culture. Nature 1977; 267:531-2

112. PetersonL, Brittberg M, Kiviranta I, Akerlund EL, Lindahl A. Autologous chondrocyte transplantation. Biomechanics and long-term durability. Am J Sports Med 2002; 30:2-12.

113. Anders S, Gellissen J, Zoch W, Lobenhoffer P, Grifka J, Behrens P. Autologous Matrix induced chondrogenesis (AMIC) for focal chondral defects of the knee – first clinical and MRI results. ICRS 2006. Abstract

114. Behrens P. Matrix-coupled microfracture. A new concept for cartilage defect repair. Arthroskopie 2005; 18:193-7.

115. Wakitani S, Goto T, Pineda SJ, Young RG, Mansour JM, Caplan AI. Mesenchymal cellbased repair of large, full-thickness defects of articular cartilage. J Bone Joint Surg Am 1994; 76:579-92.

116. Wakitani S, Mitsuoka T, Nakamura N et al. Autologous bone marrow stromal cell transplantation for repair of full-thickness articular cartilage defects in human patellae: two case reports. Cell Transplant. 2004; 13:595-600.

117. Wakitani S, Imoto K, Yamamoto T, Saito M, Murata N, Yoneda M. Human autologous culture expanded bone marrow mesenchymal cell transplantation for repair of cartilage defects in osteoarthritic knees. Osteoarthritis Cartilage 2002; 10:199-206.

118. Murphy JM, Dixon K, Beck S, Fabian DG, Feldman A, Barry FP. Reduced chondrogenic and adipogenic activity of mesenchymal stem cells from patients with advanced osteoarthritis. Arthritis Rheum 2002; 46:704-13.

119. Murphy JM, Fink DJ, Hunziker EB, Barry FP. Stem-cell therapy in caprine model of osteoarthritis. Arthritis Rheum 2003; 48:3464-74.

120. Muller P, Pfeiffer P, Koglin J et al. Caridiomyocytes of noncardiac origin in myocardial biopsies of human transplanted hearts. Circulation 2002; 106:31-5.

121. Janssens S, Dubois C, Bogaert J et al. Autologous bone marrow-derived stem-cell transfer in patients with ST-segment elevation myocardial infarction: double-blind, randomised controlled trial. The Lancet 2006; 367:113-21.

122. McDougal WS. Metabolic complications of urinary intestinal diversion. J Urol 1992; 147:1199-208.

123. Soergel TM, Cain MP, Misseri R et al. Transitional cell carcinoma of the bladder following augmentation cystoplasty for the neuropatic bladder. J Urol 2004; 172:1649-51.

124. Gilbert SM, Hensle TW. Metabolic consequences and long-term complications of enterocystoplasty in children: a review. J Urol 2005; 173:1080-86.

125. Nuininga JE, van Moerkerk H, Hanssen A, Hulsbergen CA, Oosterwijk-Wakka J, Oosterwijk E, de Gier RP, Schalken JA, van Kuppevelt TH, Feitz WF. A rabbit model to tissue engineer the bladder. Biomaterials. 2004 Apr;25(9):1657-61.

126. Kanematsu A, Yamamoto S, Noguchi T, Ozeki M, Tabata Y, Ogawa O. Bladder regeneration by bladder acellular matrix combined with sustained release of exogenous growth factor. J Urol. 2003 Oct;170(4 Pt 2):1633-8.

127. Yoo JJ, Meng J, Oberpenning F, Atala A. Bladder augmentation using allogenic bladder submucosa seeded with cells. Urology. 1998 Feb;51(2):221-5.

128. Oberpenning F, Meng J, Yoo JJ, Atala A. De novo reconstitution of a functional mammalian urinary bladder by tissue engineering. at Biotechnol. 1999 Feb;17(2):149-55.

129. Atala A, Bauer SB, Soker S, Yoo JJ, Retik AB. Tissue-engineered autologous bladders for patients needing cystoplasty. Lancet. 2006 Apr 15;367(9518):1241-6

130. Kanematsu A, Yamamoto S, Iwai-Kanai E, Kanatani I, Imamura M, Adam RM, Tabata Y, Ogawa O. Induction of smooth muscle cell-like phenotype in marrow-derived cells among regenerating urinary bladder smooth muscle cells. Am J Pathol. 2005 Feb;166(2):565-73.

131. Chung SY, Krivorov NP, Rausei V, Thomas L, Frantzen M, Landsittel D, Kang YM, Chon CH, Ng CS, Fuchs GJ. Bladder reconstitution with bone marrow derived stem cells seeded on small intestinal submucosa improves morphological and molecular composition. J Urol. 2005 Jul;174(1):353-9.

132. Zhang Y, Lin HK, Frimberger D, Epstein RB, Kropp BP. Growth of bone marrow stromal cells on small intestinal submucosa: an alternative cell source for tissue engineered bladder. BJU Int. 2005 Nov;96(7):1120-5.

133. Bambakidis NC, Theodore N,Nakaji P, Harvey A, et al. Endogenous stem cell proliferation after central nervous system injury: alternative therapeutic options. Neurosurg Focus 2005;19: E1.

134. Akiyama Y, Radtke C, Honmou O, Kocsis JD. Remyelination of the spinal cord following intravenous delivery of bone marrow cells. Glia 2002; 39:229-36.

135. Park HC, Shim YS, Ha Y, Yoon SH, Park SR, Choi BH, Park HS. Treatment of complete spinal cord injury patients by autologous bone marrow cell transplantation and administration of granulocyte-macrophage colony stimulating factor. Tissue Eng. 2005 May-Jun;11(5-6):913-22.

www.ingramcontent.com/pod-product-compliance
Lightning Source LLC
Chambersburg PA
CBHW071201220526
45468CB00003B/1106